Dementia

Types, Diagnosis, Symptoms, Treatment, Causes,
Neurocognitive Disorders, Prognosis, Research,
History, Myths, and More!

By Frederick Earlstein

Foreword

Dementia is one of the most prevalent diseases in the world today - but little is understood about it, and we have yet to find an effective cure or treatment for the many types of brain disorders that may be classified as dementia.

As of 2015, there is an estimated 46.9 million people in the world who are living with dementia, and it is projected that this number will double every 20 years. The risk of getting dementia increases as one grows older, and so the fast growth of an elderly population - due to improved health care services - has the rather unfortunate effect of increasing the prevalence of dementia worldwide.

If you or a loved one are facing the prospects of getting dementia, or have already been diagnosed with dementia - one of the best things you can do is to inform yourself about this condition, what it means, what possible treatments are available for you, and what are the best ways that you can have to cope better with living with dementia.

Table of Contents

Introduction

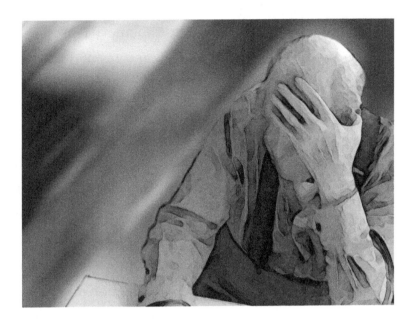

Dementia is arguably one of the oldest diseases in the world - recognized since ancient times, though it had always been assumed that it was only a normal part of growing old. We know better now due to recent scientific and medical research, and it has been determined that while the risk for getting dementia increases with age, it is by no means inevitable. In short, not everyone who grows old is certain to get dementia.

It is important to understand that some of the symptoms of dementia - and which may often be mistaken for the normal aging process - are often subtle to detect at first. Symptoms such as forgetfulness, memory lapses, confusion - these are properly considered symptoms of dementia only if they begin to interfere with a person's day to day activities. If you suspect yourself or a loved one of having dementia, go to a medical professional and ask for an expert diagnosis. This is certainly a sobering, and possibly even distressing, process to go through - but early detection may, at times, allow you to make use of available drugs or treatment that not only helps in managing the symptoms, but may even help in preventing or delaying the onset of dementia. But most important of all - proper information allows you to better accept the condition, and from there, make informed decisions about the rest of your life.

This book contains some of the basic information regarding dementia: its history, the myths surrounding it, and the different types of dementia and their respective symptoms, treatments, diagnosis, and prognosis. We also look at some of the alternative or complementary treatments available, including what the future may hold in store for dementia research.

Below you will find a glossary of some of the important terms and vocabulary related to dementia.

Important Terms to Know

Abnormal - Outside of the expected norm.

Acute Condition - Disease or symptom that appears suddenly, with marked intensity, but subsides in a short period of time following treatment

Aging - The process of becoming older

Alzheimer's Disease - Disability characterized by impaired memory and the inability to learn new material, usually accompanied by a high level of stress and acute sensitivity to the environment

Anxiety - Feeling of apprehension and fear

Apathy - Lack of interest, concern or emotion

Apraxia - Loss of ability to carry out complex movements, whether learned, familiar, or purposive

Assessment - Evaluation of a person's condition or personal needs; an ongoing process vital to therapeutic care and support

Brain - center of thought and emotion, responsible for coordination, bodily control, and sensory and information processing

Caregiver - Somene who provides care to a person with dementia

Cerebral - Pertaining to the cerebrum or the brain.

Cognitive - Related to thought, judgment or knowledge.

Delusion - The persistent belief in the truth of something that may be illogical or that is a distortion of facts

Dementia - An overall term that describes a wide range of symptoms associated with memory decline and other cognitive skills severe enough to reduce a person's ability to perform everyday activities

Depression - An abnormal emotional state characterized by feelings of worthlessness, sadness, emptiness, and hopelessness.

Diagnosis - The identification of a disease based on a scientific examination of signs and symptoms, laboratory tests and other procedures

Executive Function - The ability to set goals and make decisions

Functional Impairment - The inability to dress, use the toilet, eat, bathe, or walk without help.

Hallucination - A belief in something that is seen or heard even when there is nothing there.

Hippocampus - The area in the forebrain responsible for emotion and memory.

Incontinence - Loss of bladder and bowel control.

Memory - The ability to remember past events and knowledge

Motor - Pertaining to motion.

Neurodegenerative - Disease characterized by sudden progressive decline in the structure, activity and functions of the brain tissue

Neurons - Messengers of the nervous system

Palliative Care - Methods that ease the pain of serious or incurable illnesses.

Prognosis - The forecast of a probably outcome or course of a disease.

Progressive - Increasing in severity

Shunt - Moving body fluid from one place to another, as in cerebrospinal fluid.

Tremor - Abnormal, repetitive, shaking movement of the body

Wandering - Disorientation, getting lost, while walking in familiar places.

Chapter One: What is Dementia?

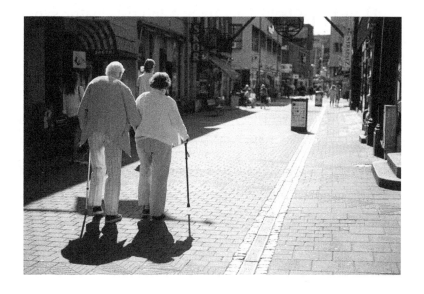

Etymologically, the term "dementia" derives from the Latin "*de*" (to depart) and *"mens"* (mind). Dementia has thus been historically considered as a condition in which a person is not of sound mind, or seems to "depart from the normal functions of his mind." It is thus a common misconception that dementia is a disease that affects the mind, often causing insanity or madness - such as when you use the term "demented." But to be more precise, while some symptoms of dementia do affect intellectual function, dementia is not precisely a disease, and neither does it refer particularly to madness or insanity.

Dementia is both a neurologic and psychiatric syndrome that covers a broad spectrum of diseases and conditions. Some of the symptoms are pretty common things such as forgetfulness, mood changes and irritability. But while many of these symptoms are indicative of dementia, not all symptoms necessarily indicate the presence of dementia. This chapter provides some basic information that seeks to clarify the rudiments of dementia: its basic definition and history.

1. Defining Dementia

Also known as senility, dementia is a syndrome, or a group of correlated symptoms, that indicate a decline in mental ability severe enough to interfere or impede with one's normal functions in daily life. The symptoms must last longer than six months, and must not have been present since birth. Such symptoms are more commonly seen among the elderly, but to constitute Dementia, the intellectual decline must be in excess of that which can be considered part of the normal course of aging. To be more precise, dementia or senility is not caused by aging per se, but by certain brain diseases. It is certainly true, however, that the risk of developing dementia increases as one gets older, especially for those over the age of 65.

Dementia is indicated by the gradual loss of cognitive abilities. And given the central importance of the brain in many of our normal physiological processes, the symptoms can vary greatly. In order to constitute dementia, at least two of the following five core mental functions must be significantly affected:

- Memory
- The ability to focus and pay attention
- Communication and language
- Reasoning and judgment
- Visual perception

The difficulties that can manifest in one's daily life are varied. Aside from the affected core mental processes, other secondary effects can include emotional difficulties such as apathy or a difficulty in controlling emotions. There may be a withdrawal from social activities, a loss of empathy, depression, making false claims or statements, mood changes, confusion, and even hallucinations. The ability to live independently is thus difficult if not impossible, as the performance of day-to-day tasks may prove problematic, and decision-making abilities may also be severely compromised.

Myths about Dementia

To further illuminate what constitutes Dementia, it is helpful to know what Dementia does not cover. The following are some myths and misconceptions regarding this syndrome:

- *That Dementia is a natural part of aging.* It isn't, and certainly not inevitable with old age. While the risk of getting Dementia does increase with old age, not everybody gets dementia. It is estimated that it affects only 5% of the population who are older than 65. This percentage does increase, however, as one advances in age. But there are still millions of people in their 80s and 90s who do not suffer from memory loss or other symptoms of Dementia.
- *That only old people get Dementia.* Dementia is not defined by age, but by the decline in cognitive abilities. While it is more common among those

advanced in age, it can also afflict younger individuals. The causes are myriad, some of which do affect younger people, such as head injuries, alcohol, and drug abuse. Though uncommon, people as young as 30 can also have Alzheimer's disease.

- *That Alzheimer's disease and dementia are the same.* Dementia is a broad, umbrella term covering various types of diseases and conditions, including Alzheimer's disease. Alzheimer's disease is a type of Dementia, but Dementia also covers other types of mental impairment conditions or diseases.

- *That people with Dementia don't know what they want and don't understand what's going on around them.* Dementia does not affect a person's consciousness. Awareness and communication are governed by different areas of the brain. Often, they *do* know what they want, and they *do* understand what is going on around them. They may simply have trouble articulating themselves or communicating to others.

- *Memory loss is equivalent to Dementia.* Memory loss is certainly a common symptom in cases of Dementia, but memory loss alone is not sufficient to constitute Dementia. Dementia usually consists of multiple symptoms in addition to memory loss.

- *If there is no memory loss, there is no dementia.* Dementia can affect various mental functions in addition to memory. Others include the ability to focus; communication and language; reasoning and judgment; and visual perception. A person who suffers from impairment in at least two of these other core mental functions, even if it does not include memory loss, can still be diagnosed with Dementia.

- *A person diagnosed with Dementia is mentally incompetent.* Not necessarily. There are different stages of Dementia, and in the less severe cases, a person can still be capable of making sound decisions for themselves.

- *Dementia causes aggressioin and violence.* Again, given Dementia's broad coverage of different types of diseases and conditions, while some can display aggression or violence, this is not true for everyone. For others, the symptoms can simply include memory loss of difficulty in communication. Though aggression and violence can occur as a result of a patient's frustration or discomfort due to the various clinical symptoms he is experiencing.

- *People with Dementia become like children.* They don't - they have a lifetime's experience and the maturity that goes with it. It is just that they become restricted by the symptoms they are experiencing, whether in their capacity to remember things, to focus, or to communicate. While they may demonstrate certain childlike qualities, they are not children and should not be treated as such.

2. History of Dementia

Dementia has its roots in the ancient world. The word itself derives from Latin: the prefix *de* meaning *to depart*, and *mens* meaning *mind*. Originally, therefore, Dementia was seen as a condition in which a person seems to "depart his mind."

Originally, dementia was of a broader definition, and applied simply to anyone who had lost their ability to reason. It was mainly associated with old age, and was treated both medically as well as philosophically, as something associated with old age. Aristotle's medical writings, for instance, considered mental decay in advanced age all but inevitable. Plato's interest was in considering the elderly unsuited for positions of responsibility, and even the characters for dementia in Chinese medical texts translate to "foolish old person."

Two notable contributions were those of Cicero and Roger Bacon. Cicero, a Roman statesman, did not consider dementia as inevitable, but "affected only those old men who were weak-willed." Roger Bacon, on the other hand, asserted that it was the brain, rather than the heart, that was the center of memory. For a long time, the Aristotelian view was dominant, and dementia was considered normal, even inevitable, among the elderly. It was often referred to as senile dementia, or senility. It is to be noted that Pythagoras referred to several distinct phases of the human lifespan, the last two being old age (63-79), and advanced age (80 and above), and considered both a period of "senium" or a period of mental and physical decay, "where the mind is reduced to the imbecility of the first epoch of infancy."

The modern definition of dementia seems to be a gradual evolution from its original broad definition to a limitation or narrowing of focus, mostly based on the identification and recognition of the different types of conditions or diseases that fall under the ambit of dementia, and their respective causes, many of which negate the presumption that dementia is inevitable with old or advanced age.

- Cerebral atherosclerosis was originally believed to be the cause of dementia in the elderly. Opinions diverged on whether this was caused by blockages to the major arteries supplying the brain, or whether it was caused by small strokes within the vessels of the cerebral cortex. In the 1960s, a link was established between neurodegenerative diseases and age-related cognitive decline.
- In California in 1913, Syphilitic dementia, also known as general paresis of the insane, or mental illness caused by late-stage syphilis, was identified by Japanese scientist Hideyo Noguchi as being caused by the spirochete "Treponema Pallidum" in the brain. This was one of the more common forms of dementia, though nowadays, this has largely been eradicated by the development and use of penicillin after WWII.
- Until 1952, dementia praecox (or precocious dementia), also sometimes referred to as schizophrenia, was considered a type of mental illness that was normal in elderly persons. After the 1920s, the use of the word dementia in referring

to both dementia praecox and schizophrenia helped limit the word dementia to mental deterioration that is "permanent and irreversible."

- In 1901, a 50-year old woman was the first identified case of Alzheimer's disease, which was later named after her treating physician, the German psychiatrist Alois Alzheimer. He made a public report of her condition in 1906, after his patient passed. Similar conditions since then were already referred to as Alzheimer's Disease. Alzheimer's disease was first included as a subtype of senile dementia, and was referred to as presenile dementia, by Kraepelin in his *Textbook on Psychiatry*, which was published on July 15, 1910. By the 1970s, Alzheimer's disease was accepted as the leading cause of mental impairment in old age.

- In 1976, neurologist Robert Katzmann sought to establish a link between senile dementia and Alzheimer's disease. He argued that much of the pathological similarities beween senile dementia and Alzheimer's disease meant that the two should not be treated differently. Dementia, therefore, is not a normal part of aging, but must properly diagnosed. According to him, if taken together with undiagnosed cases, Alzheimer's was quite common though rarely reported, and is actually a leading cause of death among those over the age of 65.

A debate then ensued on whether dementia was a normal part of the aging process, or was actually the result of a particular disease process. For a time, "senile Dementia of the Alzheimer's type" was the proposed diagosis for those over the age of 65, while younger persons were simply diagnosed with Alzheimer's disease. This age difference was eventually debunked, and Alzheimer's disease was the common diagnosis for any person of whatever age who suffered from Alzheimer's particular brain pathology. Age, therefore, was not definitive of Alzheimer's, and therefore not definitive of dementia. Neither was it inevitable, as there were individuals who did not develop Alzheimer's, despite reaching an advanced age.

Of course, the prevalence of dementia only increased recently, as humanity's lifespan also increased. Dementia is also more prevalent among women, but then women generally live longer than men.

- After 1952, mental illnesses including schizophrenia were no longer considered as falling under dementias. On the other hand, arterial conditions were considered dementias of a vascular cause, and are now called vascular dementia or multi-infarct dementia.

More recently, differences in symptoms and brain pathology enabled experts to differentiate other types of dementias from the more common types: Alzheimer's disease and vascular dementia. But clearly, dementia was no longer considered normal, inevitable, or exclusive to persons of advanced age.

Chapter Two: Types of Dementia

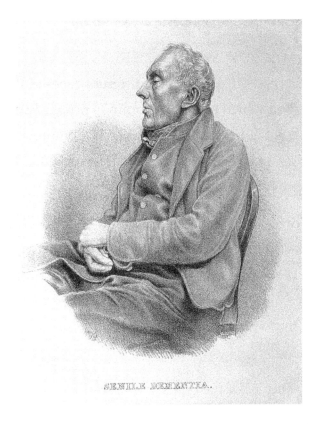

SENILE DEMENTIA.

There are over 60 different conditions or diseases that are considered as subtypes of dementia, and several ways of classifying or categorizing them. In this chapter, we look at some of these major classifications, and also at some of the more common subtypes or causes of dementia.

Different categories for types of dementia

1. Cortical and Subcortical Dementia

This classification of the different types of dementia is based on which part of the brain is primarily affected or damaged, which will typically exhibit more obvious physical changes such as deterioration, degeneration, or signs of atrophy.

Cortical dementia means that the brain's cortex, the gray matter, or its outer layer, is primarily affected. This is the part of the brain that directs our ability to process information, as well as our language and memory processes. Our reasoning and problem-solving processes are also affected.

Examples of the types considered as cortical dementia include Alzheimer's, frontotemporal dementia, Binswanger's disease, and Creutzfeldt-Jakob disease.

Subcortical dementia, on the other hand affects the brain's white matter, or beneath the cortex. Motivation, emotions, and attention are primarily affected, and can manifest as depression, apathy, or irritability.

Examples of subcortical dementia include Parkinson's disease, Huntington's disease, and AIDS dementia complex or HIV Dementia.

It bears stressing that this classification is somewhat misleading. In most types of dementia, both the cortical and subcortical types of dementia can also cause consequent damage to both the cortex and the subcortex. As each type progresses, the symptoms can eventually coincide.

2. Primary and Secondary Dementia

Secondary dementia means that the dementia is the result of another illness, disease, trauma or injury. Examples of other conditions that may cause dementia are brain infections, progressive supranuclear palsy, and multiple sclerosis. On the other hand, primary dementia means that the dementia is not the result of any other disease but is, in itself, the cause of the symptoms. The leading types of dementia such as Alzheimer's disease and vascular dementia are examples of primary dementia.

This distinction between primary and secondary dementia is important when it comes to prognosis and treatment. While many cases of dementia are considered irreversible, some instances of secondary dementia may be treated by addressing the underlying cause, in which case the dementia can be stopped or reversed. And even then, it would still depend on early identification of the cause, early treatment, and whether the condition in itself is treatable per se.

Some causes of dementia that may be reversible include brain tumors, chronic alcohol abuse, low levels of vitamin B-12, and adjustments in calcium or sodium levels.

3. Reversible and Irreversible Dementia

Simply put, reversible dementia may be responsive to treatment, either in slowing the progress or reversing some of the symptoms altogether. Reversible dementia is, therefore, a temporary condition, and may arise from other causes such as brain disease, medication, alcohol, depression, malnutrition, physical traumas or injuries, heart disease and a lack of sufficient oxygen to the brain, infections, metabolic disorders, and dementia as the result of certain environmental factors such as poisoning from gas leaks and exhaust fumes. In most cases, addressing the underlying cause can usually reverse the resulting dementia symptoms altogether.

Irreversible dementia, on the other hand, is progressive, incurable and irreversible, and eventually results in permanent damage to the brain. Cases of irreversible dementia usually comprise primary types of dementia such as Alzheimer's disease, vascular dementia, and other neurological diseases such as Parkinson's disease, Huntington's disease, Creutzfeldt-Jakob disease, AIDS, and Down's Syndrome.

Chapter Three: Common Causes Dementia

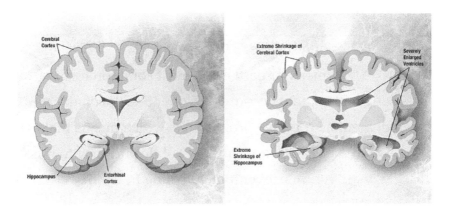

All the different causes of dementia have one thing in common: a dysfunction of the cerebral cortex. This is the part of the brain that controls memory, language, perception, thoughts and consciousness. Some - the cortical type dementias, cause direct damage to the cortex, while others may only disrupt or cause dysfunction in the subcortical areas of the brain which regulate cortical function. Depending on whether or not permanent damage is caused to the cortex, some causes may still be reversible.

In this chapter, we take a look at some of the more common causes of dementia, their signs and symptoms, causes, diagnosis, possible treatment, and prognosis.

1. Alzheimer's Disease

Basics of Alzheimer's Disease

Alzheimer's disease is the most common form of dementia, and it accounts for over 50-70% of all cases of dementia. It is also progressive, which means that even when the early symptoms are subtle and easy to miss, it gets worse over time, eventually leading to death.

What characterizes Alzheimer's is the appearance of amyloid plaques and tangles (neurofibrillary tangles) in the brain caused by abnormal protein deposits.

Amyloid plaques are clumps of toxic protein peptides or fragments, also called beta-amyloid. Beta-amyloids start out as Amyloid Precursor Protein (APP), which are produced by cells for the cellular membrane. When the APP becomes embedded or stuck in the membrane, certain enzymes snip or cleave the APP into fragments. APP fragments generally release beneficial elements for the growth of neurons while interacting beneficially with the nucleus of the cell. However, in some instances some APP fragments are snipped or cleaved at both ends, releasing the beta-amyloid peptide into space, which begins to stick to other beta-amyloid peptides.

These clumps or aggregates of beta-amyloid peptides may react with other cells and synapses, compromising their ability to function. In time, these clumps of beta-amyloid peptides grow larger. Other proteins and material become added, and they grow to become insoluble entites that are what are now known as amyloid plaques.

On the other hand, Neurofibrillary Tangles, also called tau, or simply tangles, are strands of twisted protein threads inside nerve cells. While tau threads usually work by binding to microtubules to stabilize them, should they have an abnormal number of phosphate molecules attached to them, tau threads begin to come together, creating tangles within the cell. As a result, the microtubules they are supposed to support disintegrate, and the internal transport network of neurons is damaged.

With the build up of both plaques and tangles inside the brain, neural connections are destroyed, also causing damage to the neurons until they eventually die. When neurons die, the brain begins to shrink in what is known as brain atrophy. In the final stages of Alzheimer's, the brain tissue has shrunk significantly, and the damage has become widespread.

It is interesting to note that in general, damage seems to begin quite often in the hippocampus, which is essential for memories. This is probably why memory loss is often one of the most noticeable and earliest symptoms of Alzheimer's disease.

Signs and symptoms:

Alzheimer's is a progressive disease, which means that it will only get increasingly worse with time. Medical experts distinguish different stages of Alzheimer's, and each stage is recognized by certain identified symptoms. For early onset Alzheimer's however, there are a few warning signs or early signs and symptoms to watch out for. The difficulty is that they may sometimes be confused with normal aging difficulties. The key here is to remember that dementia is not a normal part of aging. While many people do suffer from the following symptoms now and then during the course of their life, if it happens repeatedly so that it begins to disrupt one's ability to live a normal life, the best thing to do is to go to a doctor to get a proper diagnosis. It is even possible that the cause of memory loss, for instance, is not dementia, but something treatable such as medication, alcohol, depression, or simple stress.

Some of the early warning signs and symptoms of Alzheimer's Disease include:

- short-term memory loss that is disruptive to one's daily life
- displays of apathy, depression, and irritability
- a repeated inability to remember the same information, or asking the same question repeatedly
- trouble with daily tasks, problem solving, organization and planning, and other complex tasks, even though these are things you normally do
- confusion as to time and place, disorientation
- difficulties with vocabulary both in speaking and writing: exchanging names of things, inability to find the right words
- changes in vision
- losing or misplacing things
- social withdrawal, less interest in work; more time spent sitting, sleeping, or watching TV

- lapses in judgment or decision-making, such as in handling money or in maintaining personal hygiene and grooming
- sudden mood changes, and experiencing emotions such as fear, anxiety, or suspicion
- difficulty with coordination and motor functions, such as in handling familiar objects
- having less energy and drive in doing things

Mild Alzheimer's can last anywhere from 2 -4 years. Experts distinguish between three stages of this disease, and as this disease progresses, so do the symptoms. Some of the symptoms that can manifest in moderate or middle stage Alzheimer's, which can last from 2-10 years, can include the following:

- persistent memory loss, including details about his life and identity of family and friends
- rambling speech
- unusual reasoning
- confusion about current events, time and place
- may wander and become lost even in familiar surroundings
- sleep disturbances
- behavioral and mood changes
- delusions, aggression and uninhibited behavior

- physical mobility and coordination is affected, experiencing slowness, tremors and rigidity
- not dressing appropriately for the weather

Alzheimer's culminates in the late or severe stage, lasting from 1-3 or more years. The following symptoms become manifest, and round the clock support and care are needed because the person has become unable completely to care for himself.

- loss of ability to remember
- inability to communicate or process information
- confusion about past and present
- possible immobility
- problems with swallowing and incontinence
- extreme behavior and mood changes
- hallucinations and delirium
- weight loss, seizures, skin infections and other illnesses

Causes

The precise cause or causes of Alzheimer's are not yet fully understood, though it is believed that Alzheimer's may be caused by a combination of genetic, environmental and lifestyle factors. There does seem to be some genetic component to Alzheimer's, though some cases of

Alzheimer's do seem to occur without any family history of this condition. Some external factors have been identified as increasing the risk for getting Alzheimer's, and these include:

- Down's Syndrome
- severe head trauma
- high blood cholesterol
- diabetes
- smoking
- obesity
- heart disease
- poor diet
- stroke

The risk of getting Alzheimer's does increase with age. The initial symptoms usually appear at the age of 60, though younger individuals as young as 30 may also get Alzheimer's, though this is usually rare.

Diagnosis

Early diagnosis is always best, but in cases of Alzheimer's, this may not always be possible. The difficulty is that it seems likely that internal damage to the brain may have already begun for about 10 years or more before the symptoms begin to manifest themselves. The earlier the diagnosis can be made, however, will at least allow the patient to gain an understanding of his condition, to gain support and understanding from the people around him, and to make preparations. The patient might also be able to modify personal behavior of lifestyle choices that contribute to the onset of Alzheimer's, such as alcohol or smoking, high cholesterol levels and high blood pressure. Any previous head injury or trauma might also be addressed and, where feasible, might be given appropriate treatment.

In any case, at present, there is no definitive test to diagnose for Alzheimer's. Many doctors will need to consult their patient's medical history, ask questions, assess the symptoms, administer tests such as the Mini Mental State Examination (MMSE), and if possible, rule out other causes of the symptoms being experienced. A CT scan and MRI may be given that would also rule out other possible causes such as tumors or fluid buildup inside the brain. In early cases of Alzheimer's, a brain scan may show a slight shrinking of the hippocampus and the surrounding brain tissues.

Treatment Options

There is, as yet, no cure for Alzheimer's, and no proven method for prevention, although certain methods for prevention are currently being looked into. Most of it involves reducing or modifying some of the external factors that have been shown to contribute to the onset of Alzheimer's, such as medication and diet and lifestyle changes. While it may seem clear that identified external factors do increase the risk for a person getting Alzheimer's, eliminating or modifying these factors after the onset of Alzheimer's has yet to be proven to slow the progress of this disease.

The current state of treatment options for Alzheimer's fall mostly under the category of symptom management. Medication offered for Alzheimer's patients usually fall into two categories or types: Cholinesterase inhibitors that help with feelings of agitation and depression, and also support cell to cell communication inside the brain. These drugs may also help with memory problems, concentration, and the ability to cope with some aspects of daily living such as shopping or cooking.

Cholinesterase inhibitors may sometimes be used together wtih Memantine (Namenda), for moderate to severe cases of of Alzheimer's. Memantine also helps in cell to cell communication in the brain, and it also helps to slow the progress of some of the symptoms of Alzheimer's such as agitation, mental abilities and delusions. It is to be noted that the relief that these drugs offer are only temporary, and while they may help in managing some of the symptoms, even delaying the progress of the disease for a short while, sometimes they may not have useful effect on the symptoms at all.

These prescribed drugs will not have the same effect on everyone, whether in its effectivity or in the resulting side effects. Though for some, common side effects include nausea, vomiting, and diarrhea. In some instances, there might also be insomnia, dizziness, muscle cramps, and fatigue.

The use of drugs or medication are sometimes supported by psychosocial intervention such as different types of therapy. Such therapies might include having the person do activities that they enjoy, mentally stimulating activities, or supportive therapies to help the patient accept and adjust to their illness. Other possible therapeutic treatments include reality orientation, or grounding the patient in time and place information to help them adjust to their surroundings. Emotional support may also be given with discussions of past experiences and tangible exposure to familiar items from the past. The effectivity of these varied forms of available therapy do vary from individual to individual, though there does seem to be some evidence that such therapies help in reducing some of the more challenging behaviors of patients with Alzheimer's.

Finally, caregiving services must be looked into early on for people diagnosed with Alzheimer's. Gradually, a person becomes almost completely incapable of living independently, and caregiving becomes essential. If someone in your family is diagnosed with Alzheimer's, you should be able to look into the aspect of caregiving early on. Will you be hiring a professional caregiver, or will you be tending to your loved one's needs yourself? Caregiving is challenging, frustrating, and many caregivers often do suffer from physical and emotion burnout. If you do decide to take on the caregiving role yourself, prepare yourself by reading up on news and possible treatments for Alzheimer's, take care of yourself physically and emotionally to help you cope with the caregiving responsibilities, and most of all - don't hesitate to ask for help whenever you need it.

Prognosis

The outlook for those diagnosed with Alzheimer's is, unfortunately, quite poor. There is no cure for Alzheimer's disease, and one can only expect the symptoms and the brain condition to get worse with time. Treatments such as drugs and therapies cannot halt the progression of the disease, and it is yet unclear whether or not they can add more time to a person's life. Treatment, on the whole, is directed more to helping a person cope with and manage the symptoms they are experiencing.

The length of time that they have depends largely on different variables such as the age at which the symptoms started and their severity. If the symptoms began when a person is around 60-70, they can expect to live for an average of about 7-10 years, while those whose symptoms began in their 90s can usually expect to live for another about three years. But these numbers are highly variable and depend on each individual case, and some can still expect to live a long time, ranging from an average of around 3-20 years.

2. Vascular Dementia

Basics of Vascular Dementia

Vascular Dementia, or sometimes also referred to as Multi-Infarct Dementia (MID), or Vascular Cognitive Impairment (VCI), is the second most common cause of dementia, after Alzheimer's disease. The set of symptoms for Vascular Dementia often does overlap with those of Alzheimer's and other types of dementia. What does characterize Vascular dementia are changes in brain structure, and a resulting change in cognition, due to strokes and lesions which compromise the blood supply to the brain.

A constant supply of blood brings oxygen and other nutrients to the brain, and it is the vascular system - a network of vessels - which serve as the pathway of blood to the brain. In vascular dementia, the vascular system - the blood vessels - are compromised, whether due to blockages, leaks, or blood vessels that are themselves diseased. In any case, the brain does not get sufficient blood flow and oxygen, leading to the death of brain cells. This results in cognitive impairment, consisting of difficulties in memory, thinking, and reasoning.

Signs and Symptoms

Vascular dementia can sometimes happen in conjunction with Alzheimer's disease, and so their symptoms may also coincide or overlap. When this happens, it is called "mixed dementia." But the symptoms or effects of vascular dementia per se can vary depending on which part of the brain is affected. Memory can also be compromised, but unlike in Alzheimer's, memory problems are not often the early symptom of vascular dementia.

Early symptoms of cognitive impairment that results from vascular dementia include:

- difficulties with planning and organizing
- slower speed of thought
- problems concentrating, and short periods of sudden confusion
- difficulties in problem solving or decision-making
- difficulties in following a series of simple and chronological steps, such as in cooking

Early stage vascular dementia may have added difficulties in some of the following areas:

- restlessness and agitation
- unsteady gait
- depression
- sudden or frequent urge to urinate, or an inability to control passing urine
- mild memory problems
- language difficulties
- visiospatial skills, or difficulties in perceiving objects in three dimensions
- mood changes such as depression or anxiety

Other possible symptoms generally vary depending on which part of the brain has been affected, and can range from cognitive, motor, behavioral, and even affective or emotional changes. There might be limb weakness or paralysis, difficulties with vision or speech, loss of bladder control, and clumsiness or unsteady walking. Others may also display a lack of facial expression and experience difficulty in pronouncing words, a mild weakness on one side of their body, trouble managing money, hallucinations or delusions, wandering or getting lost in familiar surroundings, short-term memory problems, hallucinations, and even crying and laughing at inappropriate times.

Causes of Vascular Dementia

Vascular dementia results from various conditions that can lead to a damage in the brain's blood vessels, thus compromising the brain's blood supply, and reducing the necessary amounts of oxygen and nutrition that it needs to perform efficiently.

Various incidents of strokes or infarctions are some of the many causes of vascular dementia. It can either be stroke-related, in which case a blood vessel in the brain is blocked by a clot which may have formed in the brain or in the heart, and is subsequently carried to the brain. Post-stroke dementia, on the other hand, happens when a large vessel in the brain is permanently cut off, often because of a clot. Because of the sudden interruption of the brain's supply of oxygen, a large volume of brain tissue often dies.

One or more smaller strokes are referred to as single-infarct or multi-infarct dementia. These are mini-strokes because the clot or blockages in the brain's blood vessel is so small that symptoms may not even be noticed. What symptoms that do manifest are usually only temporary and disappears within the next 24 hours. But if a series of small strokes take place within a period of weeks or months (or multi-infarct dementia), the damage can spread all over the brain and dementia can result from the total damage taken together.

Subcortical dementia, on the other hand, is considered the leading cause of vascular dementia. This is a disease of the very small blood vessels deep in the brain, which can become stiff and twisted, or develop thick walls, thus reducing blood flow to the brain. This can also cause damage to the nerves in the white matter of the brain that carry signals, and may even cause small infarcts near the base of the brain. Small vessel disease often occurs deep in the brain, so the symptoms are usually diffent from those of stroke-related dementia, which largely affect different areas of the brain.

There are also other conditions which cause a narrowing of the brain's blood vessels, and the long term damage this causes can eventually lead to vascular dementia. Some of these conditions include high blood pressure, a hardening of the arteries, diabetes, brain hemorrhage, lupus erythematosus, and temporal arteritis.

Diagnosis of Vascular Dementia

There is no specific test to confirm vascular dementia. Various tests and assessments can, however, be administered to at least exclude other possible causes of the symptoms. An overall medical examination and assessment is given, which can includes:

- a full medical history, especially if you have a history of strokes, high blood pressure, high cholesterol, diabetes, and other conditions related to vascular dementia
- a physical examination
- a range of blood tests to exclude other possible causes of the symptoms, including vitamin B12 deficiency, thyroid disorders and other vitamin deficiencies
- brain scans such as CT scan and an MRI scan
- electrocardiogram (ECG) test to monitor the heart rhythm

- a review of medications being taken for the symptoms
- a neurological exam to test your reflexes, senses, coordination, muscle tone and strength, and balance
- an assessment of the symptoms, their progress and development, and mental abilities
- a carotid ultrasound can check whether the carotid arteries which run up either side of your neck to supply blood to the brain - show signs of plaque deposits, structural problems, or various signs of narrowing
- a professional screening for depression since vascular brain conditions are usually accompanied by depression, which can also contribute to the symptoms

Persons at high risk of developing vascular cognitive impairment are usually recommended to undergo brief tests that would assess their memory, thinking and reasoning. Those considered of highest risk are people who have experienced a stroke, or those who have heart or blood vessel disease.

In 2011, the American Heart Association (AHA) and the American Stroke Association (ASA) issued a statement that was endorsed by the Alzheimer's Association and the American Academy of Neurology, to the effect that the following three criteria are suggestive of the greatest likelihood that dementia or cognitive impairment is caused by vascular conditions:

1. A diagnosis of dementia or mild cognitive impairment confirmed by neurocognitive testing, which evaluates specific thinking skills such as planning, judgment, problem-solving, reasoning and memory

2. Brain imaging evidence, such as an MRI, that shows:

- evidence of a recent stroke, or

- brain blood vessel changes that show affected tissue whose pattern and severity are consistent with the results of the impairment documented in the neurocognitive testing

3. The absence of other evidence to show that other factors other than vascular changes have contributed to the cognitive decline.

Treatment Options

Just like Alzheimer's, there is no cure for vascular dementia. But some treatments may help in preventing further damage and in slowing the progress of the disease.

The essence of treatment for vascular disease is in addressing the underlying cause that resulted in damage to the vascular system. This can be undertaken by two ways: medication and lifestyle changes.

While there are no U.S. FDA approved drugs for treating the symptoms of vascular dementia per se, medication can be prescribed to treat the underlying cause of the vascular dementia. By treating the cause of the vascular degeneration, further worsening of the symptoms may be prevented. For instance:

- statins for high cholesterol levels
- antigoagulants and antiplatelets to reduce the risk of blood clots and strokes
- diabetes medication
- antidepressants for depression
- antihypertensives for high blood pressure

Lifestyle changes, on the other hand, are very useful for those whose risk factor of getting vascular dementia have been increased by various modifiable lifestyle factors, such as:

- losing weight
- stopping smoking
- cutting down on alcohol

- eating healthy
- regular exercise
- monitoring blood pressure, cholesterol, and blood sugar levels and keeping them within recommended limits

On a more positive note, introducing affirmative and healthy lifestyle changes may also prove beneficial, such as stress management and mentally stimulating activities. One can also create a network of support, within a professional therapeutic environment if necessary, and this can help in one's acceptance of their condition, as well as their ability to communicate to others, including family and loved ones, their feelings and thoughts about their condition.

Prognosis

The prognosis for vascular dementia is thought to be worse than that of Alzheimer's, ranging from about 3-5 years. This is probably because while Alzheimer's advances at a slow and steady rate of deterioration, the onset of vascular dementia can be sudden and might even be the direct cause of death when the blood supply to the brain is interrupted. The causes of death might be a stroke, heart disease, or an infection.

There might be periods, however, when the symptoms might seem to improve, especially when the person undergoes medication and therapy to treat any physical incapacity and to stimulate his mental functioning. If another stroke happens, however, more brain function can be compromised.

Arguably the best possible treatment for vascular dementia at this time is early diagnosis and immediate treatment by medication, appropriate therapy, and risk reduction by lifestyle changes. In this way, further damage can be prevented, halted, or sometimes even reversed.

3. Dementia with Lewy Bodies (DLB)

Basics of Dementia with Lewy Bodies

Dementia with Lewy Bodies is a type of dementia that shares some of the symptoms of Alzheimer's disease and Parkinson's disease. It is also sometimes called Lewy Body dementia (LBD), diffuse Lewy body disease, cortical Lewy body disease, and senile dementia of the Lewy type.

Lewy bodies were named after Frederick H. Lewy, M.D., a neurologist who worked in Dr. Alois Alzheimer's laboratory in the early 1900s, and was the one who discovered the brain abnormalities whose main component is the alpha-synuclein protein. While alpha-synuclein proteins are found widely in the brain, their function is as yet unknown. Abnormal deposits of this protein are referred to as Lewy bodies, and while their contribution to dementia is still unclear, studies show a link between their presence and the loss of connection between nerve cells.

It is to be noted that Lewy bodies are also present in Parkinson's disease, and together with DLB, they are referred to as Lewy body disorders. This is probably why many of their symptoms are similar and overlapping. Some physicians even use the two terms interchangeably to refer to the same condition. What does distinguish them seems to depend on which set of symptoms appeared first. If motor and movement changes occurred at least a year before cognitive decline, it is identified as Parkinson's disease. But if mobility symptoms appeared at the same time with cognitive decline, then it is diagnosed as Dementia with Lewy bodies. It seems that Parkinson's disease refers primarily to the loss of motor control exclusively, with symptoms such as weakness and tremors and rigidity, while DLB is characterized by the presence of cognitive decline in addition to other physical symptoms. The difficulty is that those who are diagnosed with Parkinson's disease may later on develop dementia, which further blurs the line between the two conditions. Of course, sometimes it may take as long as 10 to 15 years before dementia develops, after the initial diagnosis of Parkinson's disease. It is estimated that only about 20% of people diagnosed with Parkinson's disease later develop dementia.

The primary culprit in DLB, in any case - the protein deposits referred to as Lewy bodies - are present in both cases, and it seems that the difference in symptoms mainly depend on the part of the brain that is affected.

Signs and Symptoms

There is a great overlap of many of the symptoms of the different types of dementia, and many medical experts believe that DLB is an under-diagnosed condition because it is usually diagnosed as something else. Post-examination of the brain cells confirm the presence of DLB, and it is theorized that it may actually account for as much as 10% of all dementia cases.

Similar to Alzheimer's, the initial symptoms may be subtle though there will be a gradual progression. The signs and symptoms are varied, and DLB has many symptoms common to both Alzheimer's and Parkinson's disease, such as visiospatial difficulties, depression, and fluctuating cognitive difficulties that manifest as difficulties with memory, planning and organizing and problems with alertness and attention. The effect on memory is usually of a lesser degree in DLB compared to Alzheimer's, especially during the initial stages of DLB.

Motor difficulties may be experienced, similar to those diagnosed with Parkinson's disease, though the tremors may be less common. Other symptoms similar to Parkinson's are slower movement, a hunched posture, rigid muscles and balance problems. Such motor problems may sometimes cause fainting, falls and unsteadiness.

Some of the other telling symptoms of DLB include:

- Hallucinations, whether visual or auditory, such as seeing things that are not there, hearing things that are not real, which are often experienced as detailed and very convincing. It is estimated that about 75% of people with LBD suffer from recurrent visual hallucinations.
- Delusions may occur because of the combination of visual difficulties and hallucinations, and a person may end up believing things that are not true, such as thinking that there are strangers living in the house, that a family member may have been

replaced by an impostor, or that they are being persecuted.

- Visual difficulties, such as double vision, or minsterpretation of what they see
- Rapid Eye Movement (REM) sleep behavior disorder, or sometimes referred to as RBD. This includes vivid and persistent dreams, falling out of bed, purposeful or violent movements as they try to act out nightmares. A person may sleep easily during the day but have disturbed or restless nights.

As DLB progresses, the symptoms do become worse over time. The decline of memory and cognitive abilities begin to resemble that of middle or late-stage Alzheimer's, and people may also develop extreme behavioral changes such as restlessness, agitation, or shouting out.

Causes of DLB

The causes of DLB are not fully understood, but because of its sporadic appearance, it does not seem to have any strong hereditary or genetic links. Those who are diagnosed with DLB have no clear family history of the disease.

DLB affects men and women about equally, and is more commonly seen among those over the age of 65, though younger people may also develop DLB. Risk factors that increase the chances of developing DLB are similar to the risk factors of most types of dementia, including conditions such as diabetes, high blood pressure, high cholesterol levels, and lifestyle factors such as smoking, alcohol and unhealthy diets. Head injuries or head trauma may also be a contributory factor.

Diagnosis for DLB

DLB is a difficult condition to diagnose, particularly because of its similarity to other conditions. In its early stages, it is often mistaken for Alzheimer's disease and/or vascular dementia. Generally, however, LBD tends to progress more rapidly than Alzheimer's, and decline can take place in the first few months. It is recommended that if LBD is suspected, diagnosis should ideally be made by a specialist with an experience of this condition. It is crucial that proper diagnosis of DLB should be made because people who suffer from this disease are often hypersensitive to certain medication. Early diagnosis can benefit patients because appropriate treatment may improve their lives significantly. On the other hand, they may also react negatively with the wrong type of drugs.

Diagnosis is usually made from a series of tests and examinations, including:

- the person's medical history, including the onset and progress of their symptoms
- a neurological test of their balance and reflexes
- a cognitive test is sometimes administered, though this can be complicated by visual difficultis and the sporadic and intermittent nature of DLB
- brain scans can help to clarify the diagnosis, and a CT and MRI scan can rule out other causes such as a brain tumor or vascular dementia. A reduced density of dopamine nerve cells at the base of the brain ay help to confirm a DLB diagnosis.

As with most types of dementia, diagnosis is only clinical, or an expression of the doctor's best professional judgment based on the symptoms and test results. In general though, DLB is found when both dementia and movement symptoms are present, and where the dementia symptoms occurred first, taking place at least a year before the appearance of movement symptoms.

Treatment Options

There is no cure for LBD, and any treatment options currently offered usually work only by addressing the symptoms.

Drug or medical treatment of DLB, however, is quite complicated. Individuals react differently to medication, and it would seem that in some instances, antipsychotic drugs may have a negative effect on movement, while treatment of movement and cognitive difficulties may worsen psychosis and halluciation. A careful balance must be struck, and it is important to remain flexible in what works and what doesn't. On the other hand, other forms of medication, such as those used for urinary incontinence and even antihistamines may only worsen their condition.

LBD patients typically show a hypersensitivity to certain medication, and experts usually advise against it. When available, non-drug options are usually advised first. These can include:

- supportive treatments such as therapy to help improve movement difficulties, language and communication abilities, and their ability to handle everyday tasks

- cognitive exercises and psychological therapies canhelp with memory loss, disorientation and confusion
- caregiving options are advisable because a person diagnosed with DLB may have difficulty managing their daily routines and tasks, and selected caregivers must be able to handle the day to day changes in mental, emotional and behavioral symptoms, as well as the how best to handle delusions or hallucinations

Prognosis

Eventually, someone diagnosed with DLB is likely to need extensive care. The rate of progression and life expectancy is variable, but on the average, a person can live for about 5-8 years after the first symptoms have appeared.

4. Frontotemporal Dementia

Basics of Frontotemporal Dementia

Also referred to as FTD, Frontotemporal dementia was originally called "Pick's Disease," after Arnold Pick, the physician who first described a patient with distinct symptoms of this condition, particularly affecting language. Some physicians still do use the term Pick's Disease.

FTD refers to a group of diverse disorders that primarily affect the frontal and temporal lobes of the brain - which are primarily associated with personality, behavior and language. Dramatic changes in these areas comprise the different symptoms of those diagnosed with FTD. Muscle and motor controls may also be affected.

Of the various diseases that fall under the category of FTD, there are three recognized subtypes:

1. Behavior variant frontotemporal dementia (bvFTD)

2. Primary progressive aphasia (PPA)

3. Disturbances of motor (movement or muscle) function.

These three subtypes affect behavior (personality changes); language skills (writing, speaking and comprehension); and muscle or motor functions, respectively. Often misdiagnosed as Alzheimer's or as a psychiatric condition, FTD can occur at a younger age, generally between the ages of 40 and 75.

Signs and Symptoms

Despite the similarities of the symptoms of FTD with Alzheimer's, there are key differences which can help to distinguish the two. FTD usually occurs at a younger age than Alzheimer's, and memory loss, confusion or getting lost in familiar surroundings, and hallucinations and delusions are more common in Alzheimer's. In FTD, the following are some of the distinct symptoms that can manifest in a person, and are usually more prominent:

- prominent or dramatic behavioral changes that can affect their personality, interpersonal relationships and conduct, including their capacity for judgment, empathy and foresight, and poor impulse control
- problems with speech, such as losing the ability to formulate words or sentences, or labored and ungrammatical speaking; this may sometimes be referred to as Semantic Dementia (SD)
- Amyotrophic lateral sclerosis (ALS), or Lou Gehrig's disease, which causes muscle weakness
- Corticobasal syndrome, which causes stiffness and lack of coordiantion in the arms and legs
- Progressive supranuclear Palsy (PSP) which causes abnormal eye movements, muscle stiffness, a difficulty in walking, and posture changes
- compulsive behaviors that are usually related to abnormal eating behavior

- cognitive deterioration in terms of planning and organizing

These symptoms are mainly classified according to the respective functions of the frontal and temporal lobes. In contrast to other types of dementia, particularly Alzheimer's, the perception, memory and spatial skills are often preserved.

Causes of FTD

What causes FTD are in essence similar to other types of dementia: an unusual buildup of protein in the brain. There are two types of protein buildup involved in FTD: the protein tau, and the protein TDP-43. Microscopic and abnormal protein-filled structures referred to as Pick's bodies, develop within the brain cells. These two types of abnormal protein buildup seem to affect primarily the frontal and temporal lobes of the brain, though the reason for this is unclear. These two affected areas eventually shrink over time.

There does seem to be a genetic link to FTD. Up to 40% of those diagnosed have a family history of this condition. There are no known risk factors aside from a family history or a similar disorder, though some experts assume taht medical and lifestyle factors are also contributory factors.

Diagnosis of FTD

Diagnosis of FTD is not easy. For one thing, it is not as common as other types of dementia such as Alzheimer's and Vascular Dementia. For another, since FTD usually occurs at an earlier age, and memory changes are not a prominent symptom, experts may not initially suspect dementia. The great variation of its symptoms may also be diagnosed as something else, such as Alzheimer's, depression, schizophrenia, or obsessive-compulsive disorders. Sometimes, language or memory problems may be misdiagnosed as the result of a stroke. The difficulty is compounded because sometimes, early stages of FTD may reveal brain scans that often appear normal.

There is no direct test to screen for FTD, and diagnosis is usually the result of various tests including a general physical examination, assessment of one's family history, cognitive abilities, and the history of their specific symptoms. Blood tests, brain scans, and an assessment of a person's cognitive abilities may also be conducted. If a genetic variant is strongly suspected, genetic testing may confirm the diagnosis.

In recent years, new criteria to diagnose bvFTD or behavioral FTD have been developed, at least three of which must be present for a clinical diagnosis. These include:

1. Disinhibition
2. Apathy/Inertia
3. Loss of Sympathy/Empathy
4. Perseverative/Compulsive behaviors
5. Hyperorality
6. Dysexecutive neuropsychological profile

There have also been some interest in the use of certain neuropsychological tests that monitor a person's decision-making abilities and their ability to monitor their own behavior. These types of tests, particularly the Iowa gambling task and the Faux Pas Recognition test, have been found to be sensitive to changes or dysfunctions in the orbitofrontal cortex, where early brain degeneration happens. These tests have been seen to be important alternatives for diagnostic testing because MRI scans cannot usually detect early degeneration.

More recent developments have combined five different tests including those mentioned above into a more comprehensive and frontal lobe degeneration-specific testing, and is now known as the Executive and Social Cognition Battery neuropsychological testing. This has been found to be more sensitive to early stages of behavioral FTD.

Treatment Options

FTD is progressive, and the symptoms usually grow worse with time. While there are no specific treatments for FTD per se, medication can address some of the symptoms such as depression, irritability and depression. Disinhibition and compulsive behaviors may also be managed with the use of prescribed medication.

Therapy can help people adapt to the gradual loss of their speech and motor functions. Caregiving and social support may also be needed, as there might be displays of rude and insulting behavior, and a lack of empathy and concern for others. Family and even work environments may be significantly affected, especially since FTD occurs at an earlier age.

Prognosis

Severe FTD results in muscle weakness and problems with coordination, and persons diagnosed can be bound to a bed or a wheelchair. Difficulties with muscular control can cause problems in swallowing, chewing and bladder or bowel control, and death can result from urinary tract or lung infection. A person diagnosed with FTD can live for an average of about 8-10 years after the symptoms have appeared.

Chapter Four: Other Causes of Dementia

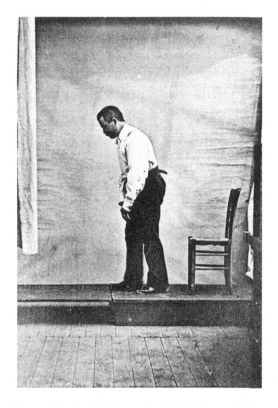

Because of the relatively broad definition of dementia as referring to "brain-related illnesses or conditions which cause cognitive decline more severe than that which occurs during the normal course of aging," it is difficult to provide a comprehensive and exhaustive list of what, precisely, constitutes dementia. The symptoms themselves are so varied and diverse that they can occur in many other types of illnesses, which, while not necessarily classified as dementia, may at least be considered as conditions leading to dementia or dementia-like symptoms.

There have been identified other possible causes of dementia, though they are considerably more rare in occurrence. This chapter provides a brief overview of some of these uncommon or infrequent causes of dementia.

1. Progressive Supranuclear Palsy (PSP)

PSP is also sometimes referred to as Steele-Richardson-Olszewski syndrome, after the physicians who described the condition back in 1963. This condition mainly affects walking, balance and eye movements.

Many of the symptoms of PSP are similar to those of Parkinson's disease, and is often misdiagnosed as such. Some of the distinctive PSP symptoms include muscle stiffness, an inability to walk, and dizziness which can result in fainting spells. The person might also experience moments of forgetfulness, personality changes, and a loss of interest that can result in social withdrawal.

In the later stages of PSP, there might be visual problems such as difficulty in controling eye movements, "tunnel vision," and gaze dysfunction. They may also suffer from some mental or cognitive problems, though these usually range from mild to moderate. Typical examples are a slowing of thought processes and a difficulty in thinking and analyzing problems.

Other possible symptoms that may be experienced include headaches, fatigue, dizziness, depression, slower movement, facial stiffness, slurred speech, and a mild shaking of the hands.

While PSP is not considered to be genetic, research shows that there may be a genetic predisposition which can be inherited, and which can make some more susceptible to this disease.

There is no cure for PSP, but medication may be prescribed that can treat or help curb some of the symptoms.

2. Corticobasal Degeneration (CBD)

CBD is a rare and progressive neurodegenerative disease that can sometimes be misdiagnosed as Parkinson's disease, progressive supranuclear palsy, or dementia with Lewy bodies - mainly because of the similarity of the symptoms.

This usually affects people in the ages of 50-70, and seems to be more prevalent among women - though both men and women have been diagnosed with CBD. While the precise cause of this disease is unclear, there is essentially nerve cell loss and atrophy of multiple areas of the brain, including the cerebral cortex and the basal ganglia. It seems that neuronal degeneration and depigmentation in the substantia nigra of the midbrain - or the gray matter portion of the basal ganglia - occurs as a result of a buildup of the protein tau.

While some genetic link has been found, the genetic factor does not seem significant to constitute a risk factor. Symptoms can manifest in the deterioration of cognition and motor faculties, the latter initially affecting only one side of a person's body (unilateral) - though as the disease progresses, it can eventually affect both sides of the body. This is also referred to as an asymmetric onsest of symptoms. The rate of progress is variable depending on the person affected.

Some of the cognitive symptoms are very similar to those found in patients diagnosed with frontotemporal dementia or Alzheimer's disease. Many individuals also suffer from personality changes such as repetitive and/or compulsive behavior, difficulties with language and analytical processes, and memory problems. But it isn't usually until motor difficulties manifest that a diagnosis of CBD is considered.

The key clinical features of CBD include:

- akinesis/bradykinesia: slowness of movements
- rigidity
- tremors
- abnormal posture of the extremities, or limb dystonia
- alien hand syndrome, or a lack of control of the movement of a hand or arm, or the inability to recognize the actions of his hand
- apraxia, which is an inability or difficulty in handling familiar objects
- difficulty with simple mathematical calculations
- and visual-spatial impairment, or a difficulty in orienting objects in space
- numbness, or sometimes a jerking of the fingers or hand

CBD is expected to progress for about 6-8 years, gradually diminishing a person's capacity to live on independently. Like with many other types of dementia, there is no cure, and it seems that the symptoms can be resistant or nonresponsive to either drugs or therapy. Management of the symptoms is, in many cases, the best option.

Death usually results from pneumonia or other complications such as infections or a blood clot in a major blood vessel.

3. Huntington's Disease

Huntington's Disease (HD) is a genetic neurodegerative disorder that occurs fairly early in a person's life. A person may develop symptoms as early as in their 30s or 40's, sometimes even before the age of 20, when it is then referred to as juvenile Huntington's disease.

HD is caused by an autosomal dominant mutation in a gene called Huntingtin. This causes an abnormal protein development which damages brain cells. The mutant Huntingtin protein is a trinucleotide repeat disorder, and when the repeated section of the gene exceeds the normal range, it results in an excess or mutant gene that becomes toxic fragments that accumulate in neurons, speeding up their rate of decay.

This expanded gene is dominant, and when passed on to a person's offspring, there is a 50-50 chance that the children will get the disease. If both parents have the expanded gene, then the risk rate rises to 75%. While HD can affect the entire brain, it has been found that the basal ganglia - which plays a key role in movement and behavior control - are more vulnerable.

This condition was originally called Huntington's chorea. Chorea is the Greek word for dancing, and it was named thus because of the involuntary movements that can sometimes look like jerky dancing. This is one of the most distinctive symptoms of HD, though by no means exclusive. It often starts out as a general kind of restlessness, lack of coordination, and small uncompleted motions. More obvious motor dysfunction can begin to manifest in about three years. Psychomotor skills are affected, and will eventually affect general capacity of movement, including chewing, swallowing, speaking, and balance. The consequently difficulty of eating may eventually lead to weight loss and malnutrition.

Prior to these obvious physical symptoms, there may have already manifested some cognitive and behavioral symptoms such as irritatibility, obsessive compulsiveness, depression, apathy, or anxiety. As the disease progresses, there may be memory difficulties, egocentrism, compulsive behavior, speech difficulties. The symptoms are, in general, similar to those of Parkinson's and Alzheimer's. In the more severe stages of HD, a person is unable even to walk and speak, and becomes completely dependent on others. Death usually results from complications, and not the disease itself. Those diagnosed with Huntington's can usually live an average of 10-15 years after the first symptoms appear.

Genetic testing can confirm a diagnosis of HD, and some who suspect themselves to be carriers of the mutant gene take this test in order to better plan for their future. This is a personal choice, however, and some choose not to undergo the test, especially since there is still no cure or preventive treatment. Experts recommend counselling for those who are considering taking the genetic test, to enable them to make informed decisions and to have a proper understanding of the possible outcome.

Most of the treatment options available at this time include medication that mainly address the symptoms of HD, though there can be side-effects which does not make it preferable for everyone diagnosed with this condition. There are plenty of HD support groups, however, that work to spread news and information and offer a network of resources to those who need help and assistance.

4. Creutzfeldt-Jakob disease (CJD)

CJD is a rare but degenerative, and usually fatal, brain disorder. It is estimated to affect 1 in 1 million each year, and is often referred to as a human form of mad cow disease.

The disease results from prions, which are abnormally folded proteins which can increase or multiply exponentially, causing a large quantity of insoluble proteins that can disrupt neuron functions and cause cell death. CJD is one form of neurodegenerative diseases referred to as prion diseases, and are transmissible. It can be hereditary, sporadic, or acquired - the latter being caused by exposure to infected brain or nervous system tissue, usually through medical procedures. There is no evidence that it CJD is contagious through casual contact, but worldwide regulations have been put in place to safeguard against its transmission through blood donations or transfusions. A variant form of CJD may also be acquired through the consumption of meat that has the bovine form of this disease: the "mad cow disease," or bovine spongiform encephalopathy (BSE).

CJD is characterized by a rapidly progressive dementia, which includes personality changes, memory loss, and hallucinations. There may also be depression, paranoia, and obsessive-compulsive symptoms. Physical manifestations can also appear, such as balance and coordination problems, rigidity, speech impairment, and seizures.

Because the progress of this disease is rapid, a person diagnosed can die within six months after the symptoms first appeared, though there are some who can live for 2-4 years, mainly due to the slow development of the physical symptoms. Death is usually caused by infections which they contract because of the vulnerable condition that results from the symptoms.

There is no cure for CJD, and most of the treatment available aims to relieve the symptoms experienced by persons diagnosed with CJD.

5. HIV-Associated Neurocognitive Disorder (HAND)

These are neurocognitive disorders associated with AIDs and HIV infections. Sometimes also referred to as HIV-associated dementia (HAD), or AIDS dementia complex (ADC), this is a broad reference to various difficulties that people experience in their memory, mood, cognitive abilities, and physical functions and coordination - as a result of HIV infection. Some consider this as the result of the weakened immune cells that protect the neurons in people's brain and nervous system. Damage and inflammation can result by the almost simultaneous revving up of the immune system.

The progress of the disease is not typical, and sometimes the symptoms are mild enough to go unnoticed. There is even some evidence that highly active antiretroviral therapy (HAART) helps to delay or prevent this condition, and may even help to improve mental functions in those who have already been diagnosed. Dementia per se is only diagnosed when the neurocognitive impairment is severe enough that the person cannot function on a day-to-day basis.

The symptoms that can be experienced by one with HAND are variable, and can range from headaches, cognitive problems such as confusion and forgetfulness, behavioral changes, and movement difficulties. In its most severe stages, however, ADC is characterized by a nearly vegetative state where intellectual and social capacity has become rudimentary. But information regarding the progress of hand is still highly variable and often conflicting. Many experts recommend a focus on managing the symptoms through various activities such as:

- mental stimulation or cognitive therapies
- physical exercise

- appropriate treatment of other possible causes of neurological problems
- healthy social engagements

6. Multiple Sclerosis (MS)

It is estimated that about 65% of those with MS also suffer from cognitive impairment, though most cases are considerably less severe than those of classic dementing neurological disorders, such as Alzheimer's. Nevertheless, the effects - such as forgetfulness, cloudy thinking and brain fog - can severely hamper daily life. Many of those diagnosed with MS are unemployed within 10 years of their diagnosis.

MS happens when the immune system malfunctions, and instead of attacking invading organisms, attacks the myelin sheaths instead. These are protective insulation for neurons and helps facilitate neural communication in the central nervous system - from the brain to the spinal cord.

There is no definitive medical cure for cognitive decline related to MS, but rehabilitation therapies may be availed of to help minimise the effects of memory problems, to learn coping and compensatory techniques, and counseling.

7. Niemann-Pick disease type C (NPC)

Niemann-Pick Type C disease is one type of a lysosomal storage disease associated with mutations in certain genes. Of the various types of Niemann-Pick disease, type C is that which is associated most with cognitive disorders.

Type C is a congenital or genetic disease in which cholesterol and other lipids could not be metabolized properly by the cells. Excessive amounts of cholesterol accumulate in the liver and spleen, while exccessive amounts of other lipids acccumulate in the brain.

The onset is variable - symptoms can appear as early as 4-10, while others may demonstrate symptoms in adulthood. Signs and symptoms can include vertical gaze palsy (or the inability to look up and down), enlarged liver and spleen, jaundice in young children, slurred or irregular speech, tremors, swallowing problems, unsteady gait, and cognitive difficulties such as progressive intellectual decline and learning difficulties. This disease is often misdiagnosed as learning disabilities or mild retardation.

NPC is a fatal condition, and many children diagnosed with it die before the age of 20. A later onset of the disease may mean a longer life span, but it is rare for those with NPC to reach the age of 40.

8. Normal Pressure Hydrocephalus (NPH)

Normal Pressure Hydrocephalus or NPH happens when cerebrospinal fluid accumulates, causing the ventricles in the brain to become enlarged, causing damage or disruption to nearby brain tissue. The parts of the brain most affected are those that control the legs, the bladder, and cognitive processes such as memory, speaking, problem solving and reasoning.

NPH primarily affects people in their 60s or 70s, but it is often misdiagnosed as Alzheimer's or Parkinson's. The symptoms that manifest occur primarily in three areas: gait disturbances, dementia, and impaired bladder conrol.

The cause of the blockages or fluid buildup is unclear, and diuretics that help reduce excess fluids in the body have not proven helpful. A surgical option is available, in which a shunt, or a long, thin tube is inserted to drain excess fluid from the brain to the abdomen. This procedure has shown to help difficulties in walking, but have relatively little effect on other symptoms such as the lack of bladder control. Shunting does not seem to have any long-term benefits, however, and certain postsurgical complications are also likely to develop.

9. Parkinson's Disease Dementia (PDD)

This is similar to Dementia with Lewy Bodies, mainly because the cause is also the same: the abnormal protein deposits of alpha-synuclein, or "Lewy bodies."

The main difference with Dementia with Lewy Bodies is that in Parkinson's, the symptoms first manifest as motor changes, such as tremors, muscle stiffness, rigidity, poor balance and mobility, and a slowness of movement - enough to make a proper diagnosis of Parkinson's disease. Once cognitive decline takes place at least a year after the initial movement symptoms have appeared, then it is considered as Parkinson's disease dementia.

Some of the symptoms include:

- memory problems
- visual difficulties
- difficulty in concentration and judgment
- muffled speech
- depression
- irritability and anxiety

- sleep disturbances such as REM sleep disorder
- delusions
- visual hallucinations

Drug treatments are available to address the various symptoms of PDD, though extreme caution must be used in taking antipsychotics and medication prescribed for movement symptoms. They may have unintended side-effects, and may actually aggravate other symptoms.

This is a progressive disease, and the symptoms get worse with time. The rate of progression is highly variable among different individuals.

11. Posterior Cortical Atrophy (PCA)

PCA is often considered an atypical variant of Alzheimer's, since many of the pathological brain changes are similar. PCA is also sometimes called Benson's sydrome, and may be considered a visual variant of Alzheimer's. The resulting brain atrophy occurs in the back part of the brain, affecting vision and visual impairment.

The cause is also similar to that of Alzheimer's - an abnormal accumulation of plaques and tangles in the brain, but it can also be caused by Lewy bodies and Creutzfeldt-Jakob disease.

Early symptoms of visual impairment are referred to eye doctors, but the actual cause is that the resulting brain atrophy gradually makes a person incapable of interpreting and processing sensory information. It can start out as blurred vision, increased sensitivity to light, double vision, or problems with depth perception. More severe cases can cause other symptoms such as getting lost in familiar surroundings and misrecognition of familiar objects and faces. Eventually, this condition can progress to symptoms similar to Alzheimer's, such as seizures and jerky movements of their limbs.

Like many other cases of dementia-related illnesses, there is no cure, but medication may be prescribed that can address the symptoms.

12. Other possible causes of secondary dementia

Because Dementia is such a broad category that covers various types and kinds of brain-related illnesses, neither does it exclude other illnesses that may sometimes result in dementia, or dementia-like symptoms. In some of these instances, treatment should be addressed to the underlying cause or disease, some of which are not progressive and may even be treatable.

Some of these other causes of dementia include:

- Depression
- Infections, such as encephalitis and HIV-related infections
- Some brain tumors
- Lack of vitamin B
- Lack of thyroid hormone
- Head injuries
- Long-term alcohol misuse

Chapter Five: Stages of Dementia

Not all cases of Dementia are progressive, but most of them are. For progressive-type dementias, they are often classified in terms of stages to distinguish the severity of their symptoms. This provides both patients and medical professionals a gauge by which they can measure the progress of the disease, as well as determining an appropriate course of treatment.

In this chapter, we will look at the three stages of dementia - from mild, moderate to severe. It is to be noted that some medical professionals further subdivide these into seven - according to the Reisberg Scale, which was named after Dr. Barry Reisberg, a New York University physician and noted expert on aging.

1. Early Stage or Mild Dementia

In the early stage of dementia, a person begins to exhibit symptoms which are noticeable to the people around them. These symptoms also begin to interfere with the conduct of their daily lives.

An evaluation of a person for early stage dementia must take into consideration their ability to function some 5-to years earlier. Other variables are also considered: their intelligence, level of education, environment, and state of health.

Usually, some of the telling signs are a difficulty with daily tasks that they used to perform easily and a certain difficulty in concentrating, organization and planning. Their work begins to suffer, and there is a tendency for verbal repetition which might signal the beginnings of memory problems.

If you notice yourself or a family member having troubling lapses in memory or other similar symptoms, it is a good idea to consult a medical professional. This is crucial because early diagnosis may allow you to make use of treatments or supportive therapies that can help to slow down or delay the progress of the disease.

If diagnosis confirms the presence of dementia, the process of acceptance and planning can begin with the support of family and friends. A person may also look into the use of supportive aids such as notes, aid dogs, and cognitive exercises to help them remain independent as far as possible.

2. Middle or Moderate Stage

In the middle or moderate stage of dementia, the person begins to withdraw from social life, and their problem solving and judgment abilities become impaired. They have difficulty functioning outside of their home, and may even need help in performing household tasks. At this time, they find it difficult to function independently and begin to require care. They may still be able to perform simple tasks, but would need constant reminders and aids.

There is usually an emotional withdrawal, behavior changes, and a lack of responsiveness to others. Cognitive abilities decline further, resulting in confusion, forgetfulness, and memory loss. They may also manifest behavioral changs such as anxiety, depression, and paranoia.

It is recommended that at this stage, a person diagnosed with dementia must have finalized any legal or medical paperwork that would empower a trusted family member to act on their behalf once they become incapacitated. Close supervision is recommended to make sure that they are taking their medication, eating well, performing their necessary daily tasks, and living life as fully as possible. This would also enable any emergency measures to be taken immediately should it be needed, if someone is always close at hand. One should also begin looking into long-term care options.

The most important thing is that the person has a network of support from family and friends to help them accept their condition, while living as fully as possible within their capacity. Stress management is necessary to prevent a worsening of their condition that might be brought on by depression.

3. Late or Advanced Stage

In the advanced or late stages of dementia, a person is almost completely dependent on others. They need 24-hour supervision, not only to ensure that their basic needs are being met, but also for their safety. The require assistance in almost all tasks, including eating, getting out of bed, walking, and in terms of their personal hygiene. He or she may no longer recognize family or friends. Their motor and communication skills are impaired, and may no longer be able to walk or speak.

Loved ones can take care of their family member themselves, or they can hire professional caregivers. This will certainly be a very stressful role to step into, and the person providing care should take care of themselves while acting fully for the benefit of their patient or family.

Chapter Six: Alternative Treatments for Dementia

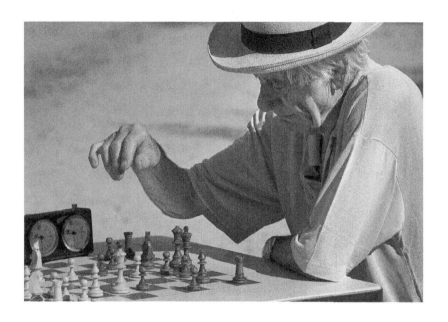

This chapter takes a look at some of the complementary and alternative therapies and treatment that may help persons diagnosed with dementia. You will also find some lifestyle recommendations that may help prevent dementia, or at least slow its progress.

It should be remembered that no alternative treatments should be considered as a replacement for professional medical advice, and any drugs or pharmaceutical remedies must always be taken after proper consultation, examination, diagnosis and medical prescription by a licensed professional. It is also recommended that any alternative or complementary therapies must only be undertaken with the approval of your medical professional, to make sure that all possible treatments being undertaken will not interact negatively with each other.

Some specific alternative treatments that may prove beneficial to persons with dementia include:

- acupuncture
- acupressure
- aromatherapy
- ayurvedic medicine
- massage
- balneotherapy or the use of water for therapeutic purposes
- biofeedback techniques
- bright light therapy
- herbal medicine
- homeopathy
- reflexology
- reiki healing

Selecting an Alternative Practitioner to Work With

It is just as important to choose a good practitioner of alternative therapies and remedies to work with, as it is to choose a good doctor or specialist. Possibly the best first step to take is to ask your doctor about any alternative therapies he or she might recommend. Discuss with both your GP and your proposed alternative practitioner the limits and the opportunities that such therapies might provide you, and how they could work with medical treatments, and vice versa.

You should make a selection among practitioners who are duly registered with the appropriate governing body. Not only will this give you a certain sense of security, but it will also help build a sense of trust with the people you will be working with. Remember that they should also encourage proper medical treatment, and be knowledgeable about the kinds of medicine or drugs usually prescribed for your condition. They should also be ready to discuss with you the scope of the treatment, the cost, the realistic benefits and effects, and any possible side-effects you might experience.

Lifestyle Changes

In addition, you should also look into recommended lifestyle changes that could help you not only in managing the symptoms, but will also help you live a full and healthy life as much as possible. Many of these lifestyle changes might seem small and insignificant things, but taken together, they can improve your quality of life considerably. It is also possible - though of course by no means certain - that they could help in slowing down the progress of dementia.

Some of these lifestyle changes include:

- Lose weight, for those who are obese
- Stop smoking
- Reduce or quit drinking alcohol
- Better stress management
- Relaxation techniques and exercises
- Cognitive and mental stimulation exercises
- Eating healthy
- Stay active and keep fit
- Get plenty of rest and sleep
- Meditation
- Work on your balance and coordination through disciplines like yoga, tai-chi, or even through dancing

- Avoid sugar
- Detoxification
- Take vitamin and mineral supplements

Each person diagnosed with dementia has a unique journey, and what works for some might not work for all. It is always best to be able to work with medical professionals and alternative practitioners who will be able to provide you with individualized treatment, depending on your unique situation, needs, and the way you respond to each treatment.

Chapter Seven: The Future of Dementia

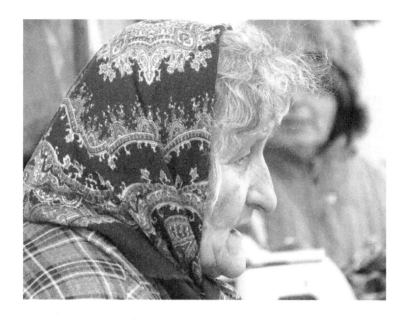

Experts estimate that the rate of the incidence of dementia is only expected to grow - the Office of Health Economics, on behalf of Alzheimer's Research UK, approximated that one in every three children born in 2015 can be expected to develop dementia during their lifetime. This is a very sobering figure, and in light of the lack of any effective cure for dementia - is quite alarming. The World Health Organization (WHO) recognizes dementia as a global health challenge, and it is estimated that there are now nearly 36 million people in the world who have dementia, with as many as 28 million of them undiagnosed.

Of course, these are just estimates, and does not necessarily paint an accurate picture of the future of dementia. Still, the numbers are such that all efforts should certainly be expended to redouble our efforts in counteracting dementia, and if at all possible, to cure this deadly condition. This chapter looks at some of the research being undertaken for dementia, as well as a look at the effectivity of current treatment efforts at managing the symptoms and incidence of this disease.

Research

In 2012, a National Plan was announced by the U.S. President to redouble research efforts into Alzheimer's and other related dementias. This is the 2011 National Alzheimer's Project (NAPA), which aims for the effective prevention and treatment of Alzheimer's and dementia by the year 2025.

These efforts are now being led by the National Institite of Neurological Disorders and Stroke (NINDS), and the National Institute on Aging (NIA), under the auspices of the NIH. Some of the areas in which they focus their work include:

Clinical Studies - to give researchers an opportunity to discover better ways of detecting, treating and preventing dementias.

Drugs - an investigation of various agents in slowing the progress of Alzheimer's and other dementias, which are now in various stages of testing

Exercise - an investigation of the correlation between fitness and age-related cognitive decline

Genetics - While some types of dementia are clearly congenital - much is still not known of many other types of dementia. Research efforts into genetics hopes to identify other genes that may be responsible, which may eventually lead to other approaches in treatment

Imaging - Clinical imaging of the brains of people diagnosed with dementia may help more in our understanding of the changes that actually take place in cases of neurocognitive decline

Proteins - Abnormal protein accumulation seems to be a common culprit in many of the different types of dementias, though not much is currently known about how they work, and why they begin to accumulate in the first place. More information regarding this can give us clearer information as to what causes them to build up in the first place, and what potential remedies may be considered.

Sleep - Sleep studies are also being looked into to determine the connection, if at all, between the sleeping and waking cycle to conditions of dementia

Stem cells - Stem cell research is currently helping research experts by allowing them to examine the effects of mutant genes and misfolded proteins on nerve cells, and to test the effectivity of potential drug and therapy treatments

International Efforts

In the UK, the Alzheimer's Society recently announced some developments in Alzheimer's research, including the possible contribution of zinc deficiency to dementia, and zinc supplements as a possible treatment. Post-stroke treatments are also being looked into.

Similar research efforts are being conducted in various other countries worldwide, including Australia and Canada.

Many of the research efforts right now are really still in the beginning stages, however, and there has yet to be a definite finding as to a potential cure or treatment. But the worldwide recognition of the great impact of dementia in people's lives, and the need for a workable cure or treatment, is leading many countries and organizations to increase funding and efforts into dementia-related research.

Spreading Awareness

Spreading the awareness of, and information about, dementia is undoubtedly an important part of the fight against dementia - especially considering the vast number of people with dementia who live, and possibly die, undiagnosed.

Many people do still live under the impression that dementia is just a normal part of growing old, and that nothing can be done about it. In fact, many of people's misconceptions about dementia can be addressed by an effective information and awareness campaign. Not only will it allow people with dementia, and the people around them, to understand what is happening to them - but it also allows them to gain access to possible treatments such as drugs and therapies which can certainly improve their quality of their lives - despite suffering from dementia.

Raising global awareness may, in fact, also help prevent a higher incidence of dementia by the identification, and avoidance and/or management of many of the environmental risk factors that increase a person's chances of getting dementia. More knowledge also enables people and their families make informed choices about healthcare, caregiving, lifestyle choices, and even family and career planning.

Index

C

D

E

F

H

R

S

T

U

V

W

Photo References

Page 1 Photo by geralt via all-free-download.com. <http://all-free-download.com/free-photos/download/old_peoples_home_dementia_woman_22 3878.html>

Page 7 Photo by Johannes Jansson via Wikimedia Commons. <https://commons.wikimedia.org/wiki/File:Aldre_par.jpg>

Page 19 Photo by Wellcome Images, a website operated by Wellcome Trust, a global charitable foundation based in the United Kingdom, via Wikimedia Commons. <https://commons.wikimedia.org/wiki/File:Medical_Times_Gazette,_%22Senile_Dementia%22._Wellcome_L0028549.jpg>

Page 25 Photo by Garrondo via WIkimedia Commons. <https://commons.wikimedia.org/wiki/File:Alzheimer's_disease_brain_comparison.jpg>

Page 63 Photo by Albert Londe (1858-1917) via Wikimedia Commons. <https://commons.wikimedia.org/wiki/File:Paralysis_agitans-Male_Parkinson's_victim-1892.jpg>

Page 81 Photo by UK Government via Wikimedia Commons.

<https://commons.wikimedia.org/wiki/File:UK_traffic_sign_544.2.svg>

Page 87 Photo by Jorge Royan via Wikimedia Commons. <https://commons.wikimedia.org/wiki/File:Paris_-_Playing_chess_at_the_Jardins_du_Luxembourg_-_2966.jpg>

Page 93 Photo by Adam Jones from Kelowna, BC, Canada via Wikimedia Commons. <https://commons.wikimedia.org/wiki/File:Elderly_Woman_in_Market_-_Belgrade_-_Serbia_%2815616229359%29.jpg>

References

"5 Myths About Dementia." Get Healthy Stay Healthy.
<http://www.gethealthystayhealthy.com/articles/5-
myths-about-dementia>

"5 Myths About Dementia." June Andrews.
<http://juneandrews.net/blog/post.php?s=2015-10-02-5-
myths-about-dementia>

"8 Dementia Myths and the Truth Behind Them." Everyday
Health. <http://www.everydayhealth.com/alzheimers/8-
dementia-myths-and-the-truth-behind-them.aspx>

"10 Early Signs and Symptoms of Alzheimer's." alz.org.
<http://www.alz.org/alzheimers_disease_10_signs_of_alz
heimers.asp>

"10 Early Signs of Alzheimer's." WebMD.
<http://www.webmd.com/alzheimers/guide/early-
warning-signs-when-to-call-the-doctor-about-
alzheimers?page=2>

"11 Alternative Medicines Explained." Laura Newcomer.
<http://greatist.com/health/alternative-medicine-
therapies-explained>

"A Brief Guide to Corticobasal Degeneration (CBD)." PSPA.
<http://www.pspassociation.org.uk/what-is-cbd/>

"A Brief Guide to PSP." PSPA.
<http://www.pspassociation.org.uk/what-is-psp/>

"About Alzheimer's Disease: Alzheimer's Basics." NIH:
National Institute on Aging."
<https://www.nia.nih.gov/alzheimers/topics/alzheimers-basics>

"About Dementia." NHS Choices.
<http://www.nhs.uk/conditions/dementia-guide/pages/about-dementia.aspx>

"Alzheimer's Disease." HelpGuide.org.
<http://www.helpguide.org/articles/alzheimers-dementia/alzheimers-disease.htm#stages>

"Alzheimer's Disease." NIH Senior Health.
<http://nihseniorhealth.gov/alzheimersdisease/whatisalzheimersdisease/01.html>

"Alzheimer's Disease." Wikipedia.
<https://en.wikipedia.org/wiki/Alzheimer's_disease#Pre-dementia>

"Alzheimer's Disease: Causes, Symptoms and Treatments."
Markus MacGill.

<http://www.medicalnewstoday.com/articles/159442.php
>

"Alzheimer's Disease: Predicting Survival." Daniel J.
DeNoon.
<http://www.webmd.com/alzheimers/news/20040405/alz
heimers-disease-predicting-survival>

"Alzheimer's Disease: Unraveling the Mystery." National
Institute on Aging.
<https://www.nia.nih.gov/alzheimers/publication/part-2-
what-happens-brain-ad/hallmarks-ad>

"Causes of Dementia." NHS Choices.
<http://www.nhs.uk/conditions/dementia-
guide/pages/causes-of-dementia.aspx>

"CBD." CurePSP. <http://www.psp.org/education/cbd.html>

"Cognitive Dysfunction in Multiple Sclerosis." Clive Evers.
<http://www.alzheimer-europe.org/Dementia/Other-
forms-of-dementia/Other-rare-causes-of-
dementia/Cognitive-Dysfunction-in-Multiple-Sclerosis>

"Cognitive Impairment in Multiple Sclerosis." Kristen Rahn
PhD, Barbara Slusher PhD, and Adam Kaplin.
<https://www.dana.org/Cerebrum/2012/Cognitive_Impai
rment_in_Multiple_Sclerosis__A_Forgotten_Disability_R
emembered/>

"Complementary and alternative therapies." Alzheimer's Society.
<https://www.alzheimers.org.uk/site/scripts/documents_info.php?documentID=134>

"Cortical or Subcortical?" Christine Kennard.
<https://www.verywell.com/cortical-subcortical-dementias-98752>

"Corticobasal Degeneration. NHS Choices.
<http://www.nhs.uk/conditions/corticobasal-degeneration/Pages/Introduction.aspx>

"Corticobasal Degeneration." UCSF Memory and Aging Center.
<http://memory.ucsf.edu/education/diseases/cbd>

"Corticobasal Degeneration." Wikipedia.
<https://en.wikipedia.org/wiki/Corticobasal_degeneration>

"Corticobasal Syndrome." AFTD.
<http://www.theaftd.org/understandingftd/disorders/corticobasal-degeneration>

"Creutzfeldt-Jakob Disease." NHS Choices.
<http://www.nhs.uk/conditions/Creutzfeldt-Jakob-disease/Pages/Introduction.aspx>

"Creutzfeldt-Jakob Disease Fact Sheet." NIH.
<http://www.ninds.nih.gov/disorders/cjd/detail_cjd.htm>

"Creutzfeldt-Jakob Disease." Wikipedia.
<https://en.wikipedia.org/wiki/Creutzfeldt%E2%80%93Ja
kob_disease>

"Dementia." alleydog.com.
<http://www.alleydog.com/glossary/definition.php?term
=Dementia>

"Dementia." Mayo Clinic.
<http://www.mayoclinic.org/diseases-
conditions/dementia/home/ovc-20198502>

"Dementia: Hope Through Research." NINDS.
<http://www.ninds.nih.gov/disorders/dementias/detail_d
ementia.htm#19213_14>

"Dementia." Online Etymology Dictionary."
<http://www.etymonline.com/index.php?term=dementia
>

"Dementia: Prevention and Natural Treatments." Dr.
Deborah Gordon MD.
<http://www.drdeborahmd.com/dementia-prevention-
and-natural-treatments>

"Dementia: Reversible and Irreversible." Lincoln/Greater Nebraska Chapter of the Alzheimer's Association. <https://www.answers4families.org/book/export/html/383>, citing Mace, N., MA and P. Rabins, MD, MPH., "The 36-Hour Day."

"Dementia." The Free Dictionary. <http://medical-dictionary.thefreedictionary.com/dementia>

"Dementia Glossary of Terms." emedicinehealth.com. <http://www.emedicinehealth.com/dementia_overview/glossary_em.htm>

"Dementia in the future: what's in store for our children?" Kirsty Marais. <http://www.dementiablog.org/dementia-in-the-future/>

"Dementia Overview." Charles Patrick Davis, MD, PhD. <http://www.emedicinehealth.com/dementia_overview/page2_em.htm#dementia_irreversible_causes>

"Dementia Pictures: Disorders of the Brain." emedicinehealth.com. <http://www.emedicinehealth.com/slideshow_dementia/article_em.htm>

"Dementia Stages." aplaceformom.com. <http://www.aplaceformom.com/dementia-care/dementia-stages>

"Dementia statistics." Alzheimer's Disease International.
<https://www.alz.co.uk/research/statistics>

"Dementia with Lewy Bodies." alz.org.
<ttp://www.alz.org/dementia/dementia-with-lewy-
bodies-symptoms.asp>

"Dementia with Lewy bodies." NHS Choices.
<http://www.nhs.uk/Conditions/dementia-with-lewy-
bodies/Pages/Introduction.aspx>

"Dementia with Lewy Bodies." Wikipedia.
<https://en.wikipedia.org/wiki/Dementia_with_Lewy_bo
dies>

"Demography." Alzheimer's Society.
<https://www.alzheimers.org.uk/site/scripts/documents_i
nfo.php?documentID=412>

"Drug Treatments for Alzheimer's Disease." Alzheimer's
Society.
<https://www.alzheimers.org.uk/site/scripts/documents_i
nfo.php?documentID=147>

"Etymology & Definition." RoseMary Beitia.
<http://www1.appstate.edu/~hillrw/Alzheimers/dementi
a%20site/Templates/Index.htm>

"Frontotemporal Dementia." NHS Choices.
<http://www.nhs.uk/Conditions/frontotemporal-dementia/Pages/Introduction.aspx>

"Frontotemporal dementia." Wikipedia.
<https://en.wikipedia.org/wiki/Frontotemporal_dementia
>

"Frontotemporal Dementia (FTD)." alz.org.
<http://www.alz.org/dementia/fronto-temporal-dementia-ftd-symptoms.asp>

"Frontotemporal Dementia: Causes." Mayo Clinic Staff.
<http://www.mayoclinic.org/diseases-conditions/frontotemporal-dementia/basics/causes/con-20023876>

"Frontotemporal Dementia: Definition." Mayo Clinic Staff.
<http://www.mayoclinic.org/diseases-conditions/frontotemporal-dementia/basics/definition/con-20023876>

"Glossary." alz.org. <http://www.alz.org/care/alzheimers-dementia-glossary.asp>

"Glossary." Dementia Services Information and Development Centre."
<http://dementia.ie/information/glossary1>

"HIV and Your Brain (HIV-Associated Neurocognitive Disorder). POZ. <https://www.poz.com/basics/hiv-basics/hiv-brain-hivassociated-neurocognitive-disorder>

"HIV-associated neurognitive disorder." Wikipedia. <https://en.wikipedia.org/wiki/HIV-associated_neurocognitive_disorder>

"HIV-associated Neurocognitive Disorder (HAND)." Family Caregiver Alliance. <https://www.caregiver.org/hiv-associated-neurocognitive-disorder-hand>

"HIV-Associated Neurocognitive Disorders." AETC. <http://aidsetc.org/guide/hiv-associated-neurocognitive-disorders>

"HIV Associated Neurocognitive Disorders." NIH. <http://www.nimh.nih.gov/health/topics/hiv-aids/hiv-associated-neurocognitive-disorders.shtml>

"Huntington disease." NIH. <https://ghr.nlm.nih.gov/condition/huntington-disease#genes>

"Huntington's disease." NHS Choices. <http://www.nhs.uk/conditions/huntingtons-disease/pages/introduction.aspx>

"Huntington's disease." Wikipedia.
<https://en.wikipedia.org/wiki/Huntington's_disease>

"Is Parkinson's Disease Dementia Different than Dementia
with Lewy Bodies?" Esther Heerema, MSW.
<https://www.verywell.com/parkinsons-dementia-vs-
lewy-dementia-98766>

"MS and Dementia Risk." Angela Finlay.
<http://ms.newlifeoutlook.com/ms-and-dementia-risk/>

"Myths about Dementia." Ellen Woodward Potts.
<http://dementiadynamics.com/myths-about-dementia/>

"Myths of Dementia." Dementia Care Australia.
<http://www.dementiacareaustralia.com/index.php?optio
n=com_content&task=view&id=115&Itemid=81>

"Myths of Dementia." Dementia Support.
<http://www.dementiasupport.ca/web/alzheimers-
disease-and-dementia/dementia-myths/>

"Niemann--Pick Disease Overview - Types A, B and C."
National Niemann-Pick Disease Foundation, Inc.
<http://www.nnpdf.org/npdisease_01.html>

"Niemann-Pick Type C." Niemann-Pick UK.
<http://www.niemann-pick.org.uk/niemann-pick-
disease/niemann-pick-type-c>

"Niemann-Pick Type C." Wikipedia.
<https://en.wikipedia.org/wiki/Niemann%E2%80%93Pick
_disease,_type_C>

"NINDS Corticobasal Degeneration Information Page."
National Institute of Neurological Disorders and Stroke.
<http://www.ninds.nih.gov/disorders/corticobasal_degen
eration/corticobasal_degeneration.htm>

"Normal Pressure Hydrocephalus." Hydrocephalus
Association. <http://www.hydroassoc.org/normal-
pressure-hydrocephalus/>

"Normal Pressure Hydrocephalus (NPH). alz.org.
<http://www.alz.org/dementia/normal-pressure-
hydrocephalus-nph.asp>

"Normal Pressure Hydrocephalus." WebMD.
<http://www.webmd.com/brain/normal-pressure-
hydrocephalus>

"Parkinson's Disease and Parkinson's Dementia." Gina
Kemp, M.A., William Buxton, M.D., and Verna Porter-
Buxton, M.D., of UCLA-Santa Monica Neurological
Associates.
<http://www.helpguide.org/articles/alzheimers-
dementia/parkinsons-disease-and-dementia.htm>

"Parkinson's Disease and Progressive Supranuclear Palsy." WebMD. <http://www.webmd.com/parkinsons-disease/progressive-supranuclear-palsy-psp>

"Parkinson's Disease Dementia." alz.org. <http://www.alz.org/dementia/parkinsons-disease-symptoms.asp>

"Parkinson's Disease Dementia." Charles Patrick Davis, MD, PhD. <http://www.emedicinehealth.com/parkinson_disease_dementia/article_em.htm>

"Posterior Cortical Atrophy." alz.org. <http://www.alz.org/dementia/posterior-cortical-atrophy.asp>

"Posterior cortical atrophy (PCA)." Alzheimer's Society. <https://www.alzheimers.org.uk/site/scripts/services_info.php?serviceID=103>

"Posterior Cortical Atrophy." UCSF Memory and Aging Center. <http://memory.ucsf.edu/education/diseases/pca>

"Progressive Supranuclear Palsy." Eric R. Eggenberger, MS, DO, FAAN. <http://emedicine.medscape.com/article/1151430-overview>

"Progressive supranuclear palsy." NHS Choices.
<http://www.nhs.uk/conditions/Progressive-
supranuclear-palsy/Pages/Introduction.aspx>

"Progressive supranuclear palsy." Wikipedia.
<https://en.wikipedia.org/wiki/Progressive_supranuclear
_palsy>

"Progressive supranuclear palsy: Definition." Mayo Clinic
Staff. <http://www.mayoclinic.org/diseases-
conditions/progressive-supranuclear-
palsy/basics/definition/con-20029502>

"Raising Awareness and Understanding of Dementia."
Alzheimer's Society.
<https://www.alzheimers.org.uk/site/scripts/documents_i
nfo.php?documentID=2970>

"Rarer Causes of Dementia." Alzheimer's Society.
<https://www.alzheimers.org.uk/site/scripts/documents_i
nfo.php?documentID=135>

"Reversible vs. Irreversible Dementia Causes." Dementia
Guide.
<http://www.dementiaguide.com/community/dementia-
articles/Reversible%20Dementia%20Causes%20vs%20Irr
eversible%20Dementia%20Causes>

"Risk Factors for Dementia." Alzheimer's Society. <https://www.alzheimers.org.uk/site/scripts/documents_info.php?documentID=102>

"Subcortical Dementias." Catherine E. Myers. <http://www.memorylossonline.com/glossary/subcortical dementias.html>

"Symptoms." Niemann-Pick UK. <http://www.niemann-pick.org.uk/niemann-pick-disease/niemann-pick-type-c/symptoms-niemann-pick-type-c>

"Syphilis History." news-medical.net. <http://www.news-medical.net/health/Syphilis-History.aspx>

"The Facts About Alzheimer's Life Expectancy and Long-Term Outlook." Kimberly Holland. <http://www.healthline.com/health/alzheimers-disease/life-expectancy>

"The Future of Dementia." Halesgroup. <https://www.halescare.co.uk/the-future-of-dementia/>

"The Progression of Alzheimer's disease and other dementias." Alzheimer's Society. <https://www.alzheimers.org.uk/site/scripts/documents_info.php?documentID=133>

"Three Stages of Dementia, What to Expect." Janice M. Wallace. <http://www.understanding-dementia.com/stages-of-dementia.html>

"Understanding Alzheimer's Disease - Symptoms." WebMd. <http://www.webmd.com/alzheimers/guide/understanding-alzheimers-disease-symptoms>

"Vascular Dementia." Alzheimer's Association. <http://www.alz.org/dementia/vascular-dementia-symptoms.asp>

"Vascular Dementia." Lawrence Robison, Jocelyn Block, M.A., Melinda Smith, M.A., and Jeanne Segal, Ph.D. <http://www.helpguide.org/articles/alzheimers-dementia/vascular-dementia.htm>

"Vascular Dementia." Dr. Laurence Knott, Dr. Mary Harding. <http://patient.info/doctor/vascular-dementia>

"Vascular Dementia." WebMD. <http://www.webmd.com/stroke/vascular-dementia>

"Vascular Dementia." Wikipedia. <https://en.wikipedia.org/wiki/Vascular_dementia>

"Vascular Dementia: Causes." Mayo Clinic Staff. <http://www.mayoclinic.org/diseases-

conditions/vascular-dementia/basics/causes/con-20029330>

"Vascular Dementia: Definition." Mayo Clinic Staff.
<http://www.mayoclinic.org/diseases-conditions/vascular-dementia/basics/definition/con-20029330>

"Vascular Dementia: Diagnosis." NHS Choices.
<http://www.nhs.uk/Conditions/vascular-dementia/Pages/Diagnosis.aspx>

"Vascular Dementia: Symptoms." Mayo Clinic Staff.
<http://www.mayoclinic.org/diseases-conditions/vascular-dementia/basics/symptoms/con-20029330>

"Vascular Dementia: Tests and Diagnosis." Mayo Clinic Staff.
<http://www.mayoclinic.org/diseases-conditions/vascular-dementia/basics/tests-diagnosis/con-20029330>

"Vascular Dementia: Treatment." NHS Choices.
<http://www.nhs.uk/Conditions/vascular-dementia/Pages/Treatment.aspx>

"What are the Different Types of Dementia?" Elizabeth Stannard Gromisch.

<http://www.empowher.com/dementia/content/what-are-different-types-dementia>

"What is Alzheimer's?" alz.org. <http://www.alz.org/alzheimers_disease_what_is_alzheimers.asp>

"What is Alzheimer's Disease?" Alzheimer's Society. <https://www.alzheimers.org.uk/site/scripts/documents_info.php?documentID=100>

"What is Alzheimer's Disease?" Diana K. Wells. <http://www.healthline.com/health/alzheimers-disease-overview>

"What is Dementia?" alz.org. <http://www.alz.org/what-is-dementia.asp>

"What is Dementia?" Alzheimer's Society (GB). <https://www.alzheimers.org.uk/site/scripts/documents_info.php?documentID=106>

"What is dementia with Lewy bodies (DLB)?" Alzheimer's Society. <https://www.alzheimers.org.uk/site/scripts/documents_info.php?documentID=113>

"What is frontotemporal dementia?" Alzheimer's Society. <https://www.alzheimers.org.uk/site/scripts/documents_info.php?documentID=167>

"What is Huntington's Disease?" Huntington's Disease Society of America. <http://hdsa.org/what-is-hd/>

"What is Huntington Disease?" Huntington Society of Canada. <http://www.huntingtonsociety.ca/learn-about-hd/what-is-huntingtons/>

"What is Progressive Supranuclear Palsy (PSP)?" <http://www.psp-australia.org.au/whatis-psp.html>

"What is the Future of Dementia?" AgingCare.com. <http://www.care2.com/greenliving/what-the-worlds-rising-dementia-rates-really-mean.html>

"What is Vascular Dementia?" Alzheimer's Society. <https://www.alzheimers.org.uk/site/scripts/documents_info.php?documentID=161>

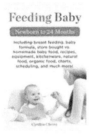

Feeding Baby
Cynthia Cherry
978-1941070000

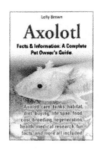

Axolotl
Lolly Brown
978-0989658430

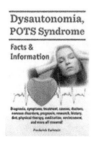

Dysautonomia, POTS
Syndrome
Frederick Earlstein
978-0989658485

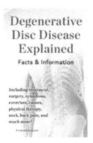

Degenerative Disc
Disease Explained
Frederick Earlstein
978-0989658485

Sinusitis, Hay Fever,
Allergic Rhinitis Explained
Frederick Earlstein
978-1941070024

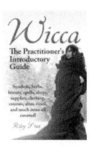

Wicca
Riley Star
978-1941070130

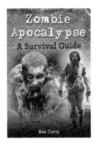

Zombie Apocalypse
Rex Cutty
978-1941070154

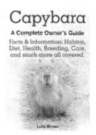

Capybara
Lolly Brown
978-1941070062

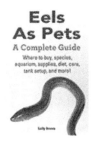

Eels As Pets
Lolly Brown
978-1941070167

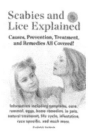

Scabies and Lice Explained
Frederick Earlstein
978-1941070017

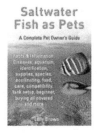

Saltwater Fish As Pets
Lolly Brown
978-0989658461

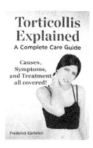

Torticollis Explained
Frederick Earlstein
978-1941070055

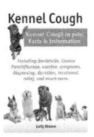

Kennel Cough
Lolly Brown
978-0989658409

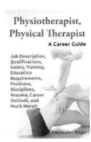

Physiotherapist, Physical
Therapist
Christopher Wright
978-0989658492

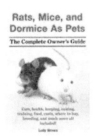

Rats, Mice, and Dormice
As Pets
Lolly Brown
978-1941070079

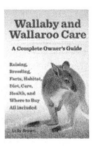

Wallaby and Wallaroo Care
Lolly Brown
978-1941070031

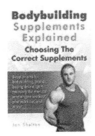

Bodybuilding Supplements
Explained
Jon Shelton
978-1941070239

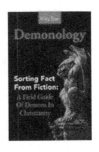

Demonology
Riley Star
978-19401070314

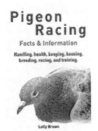

Pigeon Racing
Lolly Brown
978-1941070307

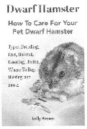

Dwarf Hamster
Lolly Brown
978-1941070390

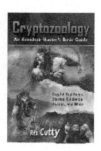

Cryptozoology
Rex Cutty
978-1941070406

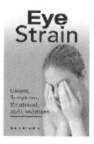

Eye Strain
Frederick Earlstein
978-1941070369

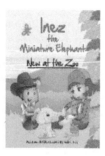

Inez The Miniature Elephant
Asher Ray
978-1941070353

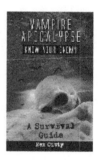

Vampire Apocalypse
Rex Cutty
978-1941070321

Made in the USA
Las Vegas, NV
24 July 2023

75164147R00079